610.72
BUD

Writing a Biomedical Research Paper

Brian Stephen Budgell

Writing a Biomedical Research Paper

A Guide to Structure and Style

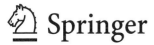

Brian Stephen Budgell
Université du Québec à Trois-Rivières
3351, boul des Forges
Trois-Rivières, Quebec
Canada G9A 5H7
Email: bs.budgell@gmail.com

ISBN: 978-4-431-88036-3   Springer Tokyo Berlin Heidelberg New York
e-ISBN: 978-4-431-88037-0
DOI: 10.1007/978-4-431-88037-0

Library of Congress Control Number: 2008938922

© Springer 2009

Printed in Japan
This work is subject to copyright. All rights are reserved, whether the whole or part of the material is concerned, specifically the rights of translation, reprinting, reuse of illustrations, recitation, broadcasting, reproduction on microfilms or in other ways, and storage in data banks.
The use of registered names, trademarks, etc. in this publication does not imply, even in the absence of a specific statement, that such names are exempt from the relevant protective laws and regulations and therefore free for general use.

Printed on acid-free paper

Springer is a part of Springer Science+Business Media
springer.com

Preface

All of us in biomedicine understand the urgency of getting experimental results into print as quickly as possible. Yet this critical step in the cascade from research conception to publication receives almost no attention in our formal training. It is as if we have been put to sea without a compass. Our collective failure to achieve widespread literacy in our own language – Biomedical Language – seriously impedes the important process of disseminating new biomedical knowledge and thereby improving the human condition. It is also a significant personal concern for researchers and clinicians in the highly competitive, publish-or-perish environment of contemporary academia. Of course, if we are clever or lucky enough to come up with that Nobel Prize-winning discovery, great science will carry the day and we are likely to get published even if our writing is fairly horrid. But most of us who publish are "bread-and-butter" scientists. We compete for space in journals which may only accept 10% or 20% of the submissions that they receive each year. For us, convincing, engaging writing will make the difference between being published or rejected, or at least it will make the difference between being published on first submission or having to go through a number of revisions (or journals).

None of this is to propose that good writing can make a silk purse out of a sow's ear. Scientific content is the sine qua non of biomedical writing. But content by itself is not enough. Style makes the difference with editors, reviewers, and readers who in their professional lives (like we in ours) have to run as fast as they can just to avoid falling behind. It makes sense that editors and reviewers are more likely to accept manuscripts which fire their interest, and readers, of course, have no use for manuscripts which they can't decipher.

First and foremost, this book is intended as a practical guide to writing good, publishable biomedical manuscripts. We will, however, also learn how to recognize and even evaluate quality in writing, and thereby become more informed consumers of the literature. Over the years, biomedical journals have published numerous articles on writing. By and large, they contain unhelpful advice which amounts to "write better" or "write like me". This guide to writing is different. Although the author is a neuroscientist, the text is based largely on the literature of comparative linguistics: studies of scientific discourse and quantitative analyses of large collections of published papers.

This book is not about biomedical writing as the author wishes it were, but rather it is about the writing patterns of successful authors, those who have published and whom we can emulate. This simple guide was written for my colleagues and friends: native English speakers (whatever variety of English they speak), as well as for the many friends for whom – as with the majority of biomedical writers – English is a second language.

Contents

Preface v

Chapter 1. Beginning a Manuscript 1

Chapter 2. The Title: Your Last Chance to Make a First Impression 5

Chapter 3. Writing an Effective Introduction....................................... 9

Chapter 4. Ensuring the Flow of Discourse: Conjunctions and Conjuncts... 15

Chapter 5. Hedging Your Bets and Minding Your Modals................. 19

Chapter 6. Writing an Effective Methods Section............................... 25

Chapter 7. The Passive Voice and I 31

Chapter 8. Writing an Effective Results Section.................................. 35

Chapter 9. The Special Case of Case Studies 39

Chapter 10. Writing an Effective Discussion 43

Chapter 11. Is It a Discussion or a Systematic Review? 47

Chapter 12. Writing an Effective Abstract 49

Chapter 13. The Process of Manuscript Submission and Review 55

Epilogue – Our Shared Biomedical Language... 61

Index... 65

Supplementary readings and self-directed learning materials to use with this text may be found on the web site of the Centre for Biomedical and Health Linguistics at

http://www.bmhlinguistics.org

1 Beginning a Manuscript

"Well begun is half finished" – or so the expression goes. In fact it is true; if we start off properly, much of the paper seems to write itself. How then can we start well?

Among the valuable advice often given to writers is to have a roadmap: to know where the paper is going before we commence writing. This advice applies both to the style and the content of the paper. With regard to the style or "flavour" of a paper, it is most important that the writer define a clear theme. In experimental papers, structured reviews and meta-analyses this most often translates into a single hypothesis which is precisely defined and rigorously tested. It is said that the most common reason for scientific papers being rejected is the lack of that single, clear hypothesis (1).

Writers may signal the direction of their paper with a very overt statement such as, "**This study tested the hypothesis that …**" or perhaps "**This study was intended to determine whether … A … or … B …**" Obviously, the thought processes which led to the creation of our research were not so constrained, but it is often possible and certainly it is very useful if we can fashion our research protocol to address one or a logical series of digital – yes or no – questions.

Observational papers and clinical reports (case studies and case series) are a somewhat different matter in that the underlying research is not structured to challenge a hypothesis. Nonetheless, the purpose of presenting the paper must be made crystal clear to the reader from early on. If the reader doesn't know why we have written the paper, how can they know why they are reading it? Consequently, we are advised to advertise the purpose of our study as early as possible in the manuscript – certainly within the abstract and, if practical, even within the title. These days, most of us decide which papers to read in full based on the title and abstract accessed through an electronic service such as PubMed. If the title and abstract don't capture the attention of the reader, the paper will not be read.

Once the purpose of the study is clear, the appropriate methods are largely evident and from the execution of these methods the results appear. The discussion revisits the purpose of the study, but now, with the new information provided by the results, attempts to answer our research question. This is the IMRAD pattern of most original data papers – Introduction, Methods, Results and Discussion. These days, structured reviews and meta-analyses follow much the same pattern. Even case studies approximate this design, but with the methods and results expressed in a case description which incorporates the patient history, examination results and interventions provided. Thus, the general architecture of papers is quite clear. Why then are they sometimes so troublesome to write?

Going back to our original premise, one answer is that the author did not have a well defined hypothesis to begin with. In too many cases, this is because the act of research was driven by the need to demonstrate a quantity (rather than quality) of research activity to some authority. In this publish-or-perish age of corporatized universities, graduate students and under-resourced investigators may be obliged to simply do what can be done with the available equipment and supplies, rather than to ask meaningful questions. Research driven by budgets and personnel policies, rather than enquiry, makes for tough writing and very flat reading. Low budget research may also allow us to circumvent funding bodies which demand comprehensive proposals. However, when we have first gone through the process of applying for funding, we often find that we can copy and paste a great deal from our funding application into our manuscript. This is our reward for having thought about our research rigorously before we commenced. Furthermore, this should alert all of us to the importance of having a very clear research question and methodology in advance of starting our research, even if we are do not need to apply for funding.

With a clear purpose in mind and the general IMRAD framework, the road becomes clearer. The International Committee of Medical Journal Editors provides more specific guidelines for content (http://www.icmje.org), and these have been endorsed or serve as a model for most biomedical journals. The ICMJE's "Uniform Requirements for Manuscripts Submitted to Biomedical Journals" are updated from time to time, and the most recent version should be downloaded from their web site before commencing each new manuscript.

In addition to the Uniform Requirements, specific content guidelines exist for the more common genres of biomedical manuscript. We will refer to these in more detail in the chapters to come. However, these should be consulted prior to contemplating a manuscript, and even at the point of designing our research, as this will ensure that our design takes into consideration the information that we will require later for our writing. These widely endorsed guidelines include:

Guideline	Research design	Source
CONSORT	Randomized controlled trials	http://www.consort-statement.org
STARD	Studies of diagnostic accuracy	http://www.consort-statement.org/stardstatement.htm
QUOROM	Systematic reviews and meta-analyses	http://www.consort-statement.org/Initiatives/QUOROM.pdf
STROBE	Observational studies in epidemiology	http://www.strobe-statement.org
MOOSE	Meta-analyses of observational studies in epidemiology	http://www.consort-statement.org/Initiatives/MOOSE/moose.pdf

If we have actually chosen the journal to which we intend to submit our manuscript, then we will also wish to consult their specific instructions to authors. An electronic compendium of "Instructions to Authors in the Health Sciences" is maintained by the University of Toledo and provides links to the instructions for more than 3,500 biomedical journals (http://mulford.mco.edu/instru/).

Key Points

1. The contents of papers are often prescribed by guidelines for specific genres (CONSORT, STARD, etc.). Hence, selecting and arranging content is not a major challenge in writing a good paper.
2. A paper is built around the purpose of the research which it describes. If the research did not have a clear purpose to begin with, it will be extremely difficult to create a convincing paper.

2   The Title: Your Last Chance to Make a First Impression

The title occupies an important place in the scientific research article as it provides the primary means for readers to locate an article and evaluate its relevance to their needs. Therefore, according to the Uniform Requirements, the title should accurately and concisely reflect the contents of the article. Titles of biomedical articles commonly take one of four forms (2). These four forms have been characterized as:

i. Nominal
ii. Compound
iii. Full sentence
iv. Question

A nominal title is a short phrase which encapsulates the theme of the article. This is the most common form of title used in biomedical papers. Examples are:
- The effect of ambulatory oxygen therapy in COPD patients with transient exertional hypoxemia
- Relationship of interns' working hours to medical errors
- The effect of an intensive smoking cessation approach on adult asthmatic patients after an acute exacerbation of asthma

The compound title is also quite common in biomedical writing and normally consists of two phrases in succession. Most often, the initial phrase is the main title of the paper, and the second phrase serves to further delimit the theme of the paper. Examples would be:

- Ambulatory oxygen therapy: effectiveness in COPD patients with transient exertional hypoxemia
- Relationship of interns' working hours to medical errors: a moral dilemma
- Adult asthmatic patients: the effect of an intensive smoking cessation approach following an acute exacerbation of asthma

Another popular form of the compound title combines the theme of the study with the methodology. For example:
- Treatment Effect of Dietary Fiber on Serum Phosphorus and Quality of Life in Hemodialysis Patients with Constipation: A Randomized Controlled Trial
- Analysis of Serum 10 Years Prior to 1st Diagnosis of Hepatitis C Related Hepatocellular Carcinoma: A Case-Control Study
- The Influence of A New Standardized Program of Neonatal Cardio-Pulmonary Resuscitation Training in Japan – A Population-Based Cohort Study

Occasionally used for biomedical articles, but rare in other genres, is the title consisting of a full sentence. While the length may be problematic, a full sentence is less ambiguous than a nominal or compound title, and so provides good service to the reader. Examples might be:
- Full-face helmets provide greater protection in motorcycle accidents than other helmet designs.
- The introduction of a standardized neonatal resuscitation protocol has reduced complications of asphyxia.
- The use of semi-solid nutriments reduces the risk of aspiration pneumonia in tube feeding.

Less commonly, one also sees the title worded as a question. For example:
- Do full-face helmets provide greater protection in motorcycle accidents than other helmet designs?
- Does the introduction of a standardized neonatal resuscitation protocol reduce complications of asphyxia?
- Does the use of semi-solid nutriments reduce the risk of aspiration pneumonia in tube feeding?

Capitalization and punctuation should be according to the instructions of our target journal. There will also be limits on the length of the title. Within these constraints, however, our task is to capture the interest of our audience so that they are encouraged to access the full article.

Key Points

1. The title of an article should be written with the singular intention of capturing the interest of potential readers.
2. There are four equally acceptable styles for titles of biomedical articles:
   - Nominal
   - Compound
   - Full sentence
   - Question

3 Writing an Effective Introduction

The introduction to a manuscript whets the reader's appetite with an overview of the paper's contents, but more importantly it justifies the investigation. Take a look at the table below which sets out the content requirements for the introduction sections of various genres of human studies.

Guideline	Content requirement
CONSORT	Scientific background and explanation of rationale
STARD	State the research questions or study aims, such as estimating diagnostic accuracy or comparing accuracy between tests or across participant groups
STROBE	Explain scientific background and rationale for the investigation being reported
MOOSE	Reporting of the background should include the definition of the problem under study, statement of hypothesis, description of the study outcome(s) considered, type of exposure or intervention used, type of study design used, and complete description of the study population
QUOROM	The explicit clinical problem [which is the focus of the review], biological rationale for the intervention [which is being reviewed] and rationale for the review

The word "rationale" appears rather often, doesn't it? Clearly what readers require is a straightforward statement of why the research was needed in the first place. This is most often worded as a hypothesis, placed within the context of what was previously known about the field. Case studies and case series, of course, represent a slight variation on this theme, since generally they don't address a hypothesis. The guidelines cited above pertain to human studies, but introductions to basic scientific papers follow much the same format, as described in the ICMJE's uniform requirements, which encourage us to:

Provide a context or background for the study (i.e., the nature of the problem and its significance). State the specific purpose or research objective of, or hypothesis tested by, the study or observation; the research objective is often more sharply focused when stated as a question. Both the main and secondary objectives should be made clear, and any pre-specified subgroup analyses should be described. Give only strictly pertinent references and do not include data or conclusions from the work being reported.

We now know what readers and editors are looking for in our introduction: background and rationale. How do successful authors satisfy these requirements? Not surprisingly (and even before the appearance of these guidelines), most published manuscripts were providing exactly the contents specified above. Furthermore, this information is laid out in a particular pattern or sequence of "moves" consisting of (i) presenting background information; (ii) reviewing related research and (iii) presenting new research (3).

Move 1, presenting background information, consists of a few persuasive, anecdotal or didactic (instructional) sentences. Because we are talking about what is known now, the present verb tenses predominate. Furthermore, there is frequent use of locative and temporal adverbials that help to contextualize the paper for the reader (3); for example, "**Between 1990 and 2000,** the rate of HIV infection **in Botswana** …"

Move 1 is also the opportunity to introduce terminology which is specific to our study area. Many journals ask that we not use abbreviations or acronyms within the abstract, and so the introduction may be used to define these components. Abbreviations and acronyms should be defined within brackets following the full term to which they apply. Once the abbreviations and acronyms have been introduced, they should be used throughout the paper in preference to the full term.

Move 2 takes us into a consideration of experimentation by introducing previous work; perhaps our own and almost certainly that of others. This move consists of two steps: the specific reference to previous work, and comments on the limitations of that previous work.

The reference to previous work includes actual citations and is often accompanied by reference to the names of particular researchers, e.g.

"**Smith et al**. reported that …" or generic reference to previous researchers, e.g. "**Other investigators** have shown that …" In these examples, note the use of the simple past and present perfect tenses when referring to single past reports and summary statements, respectively. This pattern of usage is characteristic (3). In referring to the work of others, we need to distinguish between what they may have actually done, what they said about their own work, and what they thought about their work or their field in general. These distinct aspects of reference are served by three classes of reporting verbs which have been termed (i) Real-World or Experimental Activity Verbs, (ii) Discourse Activity Verbs and (iii) Cognition Activity Verbs (4). Examples of Real-World/Experimental verbs are **associated, compared, demonstrated, examined, found, observed** and **showed**. "**Found**" is by far the most common of these as in, for example, "**Smith found that the most significant risk factor for infection was …**" Verbs of the discourse type are also fairly common and include **documented, hypothesized, noted, postulated, proposed, reported and stated**. The Cognition Activity Verbs represent only a small proportion of reporting verbs actually found in biomedical articles, and include **assumed, believed, concluded, considered, regarded, recognized and thought.** Obviously, attributing thoughts to another researcher is difficult unless they have overtly stated in print that they hold particular beliefs. Hence, reference to previous work tends to focus on what the researcher actually did.

In reviewing the literature, we will want to cite the major papers which have contributed to the conception of the present study. In general, we want to be conservative with our citations, and it is not necessary to cite multiple papers which describe the same phenomenon unless this contributes to our thesis. Besides supporting the purpose and thesis of our work, the citations will direct readers to the original source of information on which our arguments are based. The citations serve to acknowledge the priority of the work of other researchers who published before us. Citations can also draw the readers' attention to previous works which may have been under-recognized in the past, for example an older work whose importance can only now be appreciated. It is unusual in biomedical papers to directly quote a previous work, unless some critical point hinges on the precise use of words. More often we summarize or extrapolate so as to give the reader something that they might not obtain themselves by reading the reference.

The second step in Move 2 identifies negative outcomes in previous research, e.g. "However, Smith et al. **failed to** identify any cases in which…" or refers to gaps remaining in our current knowledge, e.g. "However, **it is still not known whether** the high rate of HIV infection is related to …" Both of the example sentences above commence with "**however**", and this or other contrastive conjuncts are frequently used to firmly introduce the rationale for the current study. In identifying the limitations of others' work, and so the need for ours, it is best to be circumspect. Hence, rather than "Smith et al. **failed to identify** …" we may say "The study of Smith et al. **did not identify** …" or even "The study of Smith et al. **did not address** the issue of …" In this way, the work rather than the researcher is identified as having limitations, and even this is couched in non-confrontational terms. Such indirect criticism is, in fact, characteristic of biomedical papers written in English (5).

Move 3 involves clearly stating the purpose of the current research. This may be accomplished by very direct statements, such as, "**The objective of this study was to test the hypothesis that …**" However, somewhat more circumspect statements of purpose are also common; for example, "**This study describes recent investigations into …**" Note that in this instance, the verb is in the simple present tense, as is conventional (3). Alternatively, and since we are reporting on work which has already been completed, it is perhaps less common but still acceptable to use the present perfect tense; for example "This study **has investigated** the effects of …"

Apart from our overt statement of purpose, Move 3 often includes a brief mention of the methods, particularly where the choice of methods may warrant some justification. For example, if we are studying the effects of a particular treatment on pain, then we will need methods which accurately measure patients' pain, not disability or survival. Furthermore, we may need to justify why we used one or several particular methods, and not others, to measure pain – perhaps there are issues such as accuracy or cultural appropriateness to which the reader should be alerted.

These three moves – (i) presenting background information; (ii) reviewing related research and (iii) presenting new research – characterize the introduction to the biomedical journal article and set the stage for the second section of the article, the methods section. A wise writer would approach their introduction by first creating a template based on these three moves, and then thinking about where content could be inserted most effectively.

Key Points

1. The introduction provides the context and rationale for the current study.
2. This is normally provided in three "moves" in the following sequence:
    - Presenting background information consisting of the most current shared information of those who are expert in the field
    - Reviewing related research, both referring to the work and identifying its limitations, thereby establishing the niche for our current research
    - Stating the purpose of the current research, and doing so, if possible, in the form of a hypothesis

4 Ensuring the Flow of Discourse: Conjunctions and Conjuncts

In learning a new language, we tend to think of the individual word as the basic structural and functional unit. However, in biomedical writing individual words seldom present much difficulty. Rather, it is how we arrange them that decides whether or not we succeed in creating a convincing argument.

By way of illustration, newcomers to biomedical writing initially create simple statements such as, "The prevalence of HIV infection is decreasing in Western Europe," or "The prevalence of HIV infection is increasing in sub-Saharan Africa." When advised that scientific writing is characterized by longer sentences of a more complex nature, they respond with the likes of "The prevalence of HIV infection is decreasing in Western Europe **and** the prevalence of HIV infection is increasing in sub-Saharan Africa." The writer has joined two ideas together, but would you say that they have created a successful sentence?

The resulting sentence is grammatically and factually correct (currently, at least), but the author has missed the opportunity to highlight an interesting juxtaposition which may even have been the focus of their writing. One suspects that their meaning and the interest of the reader would have been better served by something such as, "The prevalence of HIV infection is decreasing in Western Europe, **but** increasing in sub-Saharan Africa." When statements of fact, such as those above, are placed together in a single sentence, the author is inclined to assume that the reader or the editor shares their perception of the juxtaposition, and so there is no need to be overt. However, this belief may be misguided, and, in any case, the editor may be left wondering if the author truly sees the connections. Within sentences and between sentences, connections between thoughts need to be made quite explicit.

Having said that, editors may be forgiving of a weak sentence if it supports a meaningful paragraph. It is the paragraph breaks which really signal the major "moves" in our thinking and so paragraphs are the most important building blocks of discourse. Their internal cohesion, and the transition from one paragraph to the next guide us through the writer's path of thinking. Indeed, when research papers are rejected or sent for revision, a common difficulty may be with the authors' ability to construct convincing discourse, not with technical details, such as methods or results, or with physical formatting of the paper (6).

It is therefore most important that sentences and paragraphs have clear relationships, in terms of argument, and this is accomplished by the use of conjuncts. Conjuncts are linking words and phrases. While we don't want to overload the reader with unnecessary words, we should not assume that they see the same relationships between successive sentences and paragraphs as we do. Conjuncts add a little measure of insurance that we all stay together on the tour.

Useful classes of conjuncts include:
- Listing: **first,**[1] **secondly, to begin with, next, furthermore, moreover**
- Summarizing: **in conclusion, finally, overall, to summarize, thus**
- Simile: **similarly, that is, for instance, in other words**
- Effect: **therefore, thus, consequently, as a result**
- Inference: **in that case, otherwise, or else**
- Contrast: **in contrast, on the other hand, alternatively,**[2] **instead, however, nonetheless, nevertheless**
- Transition: **incidentally, at the same time**

With listing conjuncts, we must be careful not to overdo it. Consider these sentences from a basic scientific paper: "**First,** a small incision was made

---

[1] In listing, we would write, "**First, secondly, thirdly** …" not "First, second, third …" and never "Firstly …".

[2] "**alternatively**" is preferred to "alternately" which suggests "in turns"; for example, "My brother and I did the dishes alternately. He washed them on Mondays, Wednesdays and Fridays, and I washed them on Tuesdays, Thursdays and on the weekends."

in the arachnoid mater. **Then,** a PE10 catheter was introduced into the subarachnoid space." Would the passage have been improved if the authors had prefaced every step in the procedures with a listing conjunct: "**First** … arachnoid mater. **Secondly** …space. **Thirdly** …"? This pattern is in danger of becoming quite tedious, isn't it? Our writing will benefit if listing conjuncts are not overused.

Summarizing conjuncts appear within the introduction when we synthesize the conclusions of a number of studies. Hence, we see examples such as, "**In summary**, most studies to date suggest that …" Contrasting conjuncts are often used in the next step of the introduction to justify our own research. For example, "Many studies have addressed the link between second hand smoke and lung cancer. **However**, to date, none have examined the important influence of …"

By definition, conjuncts are unnecessary – at least in grammatical terms. That is to say the phrases or sentences which they link could still stand alone logically without any conjunct. Therefore, conjuncts should be used sparingly like a spice or condiment which complements rather than overwhelms a meal.

Key Points

1. Do not assume that readers and editors see the logical connections that you see in your own writing.
2. Make connections in successive thoughts explicit through the use of conjuncts and conjunctions, but use conjuncts sparingly.

5 Hedging Your Bets and Minding Your Modals

It is not uncommon to be uncertain – either in science or in daily life. Therefore, it is not surprising that we have many ways, in our writing, to convey uncertainty. Collectively, the words and phrases used for this purpose are called hedges. Examples would be expressions such as "**As far as we know …**" or "**It is thought that …**". Hedging expressions are both common and very useful in biomedical writing, and so authors should be well practiced in their use.

There are a great many reasons for deliberately registering uncertainty in a passage of scientific writing (7, 8). A parsimonious interpretation of hedging is that by being vague we protect ourselves against criticism or the territorial instincts of other researchers. If that were the purpose of hedging, however, it could be deemed a striking failure – criticism is an integral part of the process of science, and tricks of word choice are unlikely to spare us. A more realistic interpretation of hedging in scientific writing is that it accurately reflects the inescapable incompleteness of our knowledge (7). Hence, when we hedge in our writing, we are quite overtly signaling that we have reached the limit of our knowledge.

One common way of hedging is through the use of modal verbs. Modal verbs allow us to express a spectrum of probability. The classical modal verbs are:

Can, Could, May, Might, Shall, Should, Will, Would, Must

These little auxiliary verbs seem innocent enough, but they are a two-edged sword: besides helping, they often signal danger in scientific discourse and must be used in moderation. Take, for example, the sentence "Tuberculosis **may** result in death." Is the modal verb "**may**" signaling the uncertainty of science or the uncertainty of the scientist? In fact, tuberculosis most certainly does cause death in a great many people every year, and we can be reasonably sure that the writer is aware of this fact. What the writer probably wished to express is that tuberculosis does not invariably result in death; many patients survive, just as many die. In this instance, most of us are happy to give the writer the benefit of the doubt and assume that their choice of auxiliary verbs was simply an attempt to be conversational in their writing.

There are many instances, however, in which we are really left in doubt about whether science is deficient, or whether the writer simply isn't familiar enough with their topic. This especially arises when clinical papers turn to discussions of physiological and pathological mechanisms; where the writer is trying to close the gap in a line of logic by inserting a suspect point of fact. The pattern usually goes something like this:

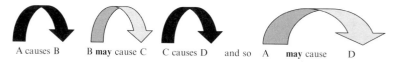

A causes B   B **may** cause C   C causes D   and so   A **may** cause D

"**May**" is the modal verb most frequently encountered in medical writing and is often deliberately used to register the author's judgment that a line of logic is not guaranteed to be certain (9). "**May**" and its companion modals also feature prominently in review articles (10) which involve the synthesis of a number of studies that seldom have completely consistent results. The use of modals in review articles justifiably alerts the reader to the flux and inconsistency in our understanding of a particular field of investigation. However, when we are writing, let's be conservative in our use of modals. We certainly want to avoid the implication that we don't have all of the available facts on hand. This can be accomplished by doing our homework and inserting qualifying statements in place of modals. In our example of tuberculosis, we can specify the death rate or describe the risk factors for death. This obviously provides better service to our readers and establishes the authority of our writing.

Apart from modal verbs, another way to signal uncertainty is to use a semi-auxiliary verb such as "**appear**" or "**seem**". For example, we could say, "Tuberculosis **seems to be** a common cause of death among AIDS patients in sub-Saharan Africa." This sentence is grammatically correct, but a cynical reader might say it really doesn't accurately reflect the current state of affairs. Some years ago, the relationship between tuberculosis and AIDS might have been in doubt, and "**seems to be**" or "**appears to be**" would have been good phrases to express that uncertainty. With the current state of AIDS and tuberculosis in Africa, "Tuberculosis **is** a common cause …" does better service to the facts, although we hope that these facts change quickly.

If hedging insinuates unnecessary uncertainty, as in the examples above, why then do we so often encounter the use of these "toning down" expressions in biomedical writing? Beyond pure grammar, hedging devices serve a social purpose in the interaction between the author and the reader. Hedging appears to make text more engaging by signaling that the author is leaving room for the reader to make their own judgment on the veracity of the proposition which has been presented. In a sense then, hedging makes scientific writing intellectually interactive, despite the time and distance separating the reader and the writer. There is, in fact, some evidence that the use of hedging genuinely makes text more attractive to the reader and even aids in the retention of meaning (7). The challenge for writers, then, is to use the proper mixture of hedging to reasonably reflect the current state of knowledge, but make the communication of that knowledge – the writing – appealing to readers.

Epistemic verbs represent quite a subtle and appealing alternative device for hedging our statements. As an example, "These results **suggest** …" is a tried and true phrase for advancing an interpretation of results without committing fully to that interpretation. We signal that we are wisely leaving room for other interpretations. Adverbials, such as "**in all probability**", "**possibly**", "likely" and "**certainly**" serve the same sort of function.

Collectively, these various hedging expressions have been termed "shields", perhaps because they shield the author from the accusation of bias. Such expressions are commonly used in the introduction and discussion sections of research reports, wherein the authors discuss the implications of their own work and that of others (9, 11). Shields are particularly appropriate when we are generalizing from the results of one study. A single study, or even a set of studies, seldom reveals an immutable truth and so we always want to be constrained in our interpretations. "These results **suggest** …"

or even "These results **strongly suggest** ..." give good service in this sort of situation. As one might expect, hedging expressions also make a prominent appearance in consensus statements (12). Such statements represent the distillation of many opinions, and commonly provide comment on specific interventions. Consequently, the authors prudently avoid definitive endorsements of any particular treatment or test. We want to be cautious, however, that we are not using hedging devices as a substitute for properly researching our paper, and having all of the facts on hand.

By the way, the WHO reports that **approximately** 1.6 million people died from tuberculosis in 2005.

That brings us to another kind of hedging expression – approximators. As the term suggests, these expressions signal lack of precision in the reporting of facts. With current surveillance methods, it is impossible to know exactly how many people die from tuberculosis, for example, or any other disease in a given year. Nor does it do us much good to have the precise figures. Where exact figures are unavailable or not particularly helpful, approximators provide one appropriate method for signaling that state of affairs. Approximators that appear frequently in biomedical writing include:

Approximately, Roughly, Somewhat, Quite, Often and Occasionally

Whereas shields occur more commonly in the introduction and discussion sections of papers, approximators are the dominant form of hedging in the methods and results sections (11).

Other forms of hedging include expressions of personal uncertainty, such as "**To the best of our knowledge ...**" and intensifiers, such as "**interestingly, ...**" or "**surprisingly, ...**". In fact, these sorts of hedging devices occur only rarely in biomedical writing (11), and most authors and editors would tend to regard them with suspicion. "**To the best of our knowledge ...**" obviously begs the question of how good our knowledge really is. Intensifiers, on the other hand, often seem overly emotive and suggest bias on the part of the author. Good biomedical writing is seldom improved by the use of such expressions.

Key Points

1. Hedging expressions signal the uncertainty which is inherent in biomedical research.
2. Hedging expressions, especially shields, occur commonly in the introduction and discussion sections of manuscripts, especially where writers wish to be cautious in generalizing from limited data.
3. Hedging is also a common feature in consensus statements and guidelines wherein the authors wish to avoid unequivocally endorsing one treatment or diagnostic technique.
4. Approximators appear in the methods and results sections of manuscripts when precise measurements are either unavailable or unnecessary.
5. While hedging is appropriate where uncertainty exists and seems engaging to readers, it should be used in moderation, especially where definitive statements or precise measures can be provided to readers.

6 Writing an Effective Methods Section

The methods section of our paper describes how the work was performed. A widely accepted benchmark for an adequate methods section is that another investigator familiar with the area of research in question should be able to duplicate the work based on the methods section of the paper (13, 14). In fact, investigations in the biomedical sciences tend to be incremental, building on the work of others who have gone before, and so other researchers will genuinely be relying on the detail of our methods section when they design and implement their own research.

Reviewers and research colleagues will scrutinize the methods section of our paper, looking for the strengths and weaknesses of our methodology. In the past, it might have been possible to conceal our methodological weaknesses by omitting information, or using vague expressions. This is no longer the case. Informed readers rely on detail in the methods section to reveal bias (in the scientific sense), and thereby evaluate the internal and external validity/generalizability of our study. Thankfully, due to the availability of detailed, genre-specific guidelines, knowing precisely what content to include in a paper does not present that much of a challenge to the average writer.

To begin with, the ICMJE's Uniform Requirements stipulate that the methods section should include detailed information on the target of our research, whether that be something as small as a molecule or as large as a human population. The manufacturers and distributors of equipment and substances must be specified in sufficient detail that other researchers can readily access the same materials. Equipment model numbers and version numbers for software must be stated. Physical measures should be reported in metric units: **meters, kilograms, liters**. Temperatures should be reported in **Celsius degrees.** Heart rate and respiration will be reported in **cycles** (beats or breaths) **per minute**, and blood pressure is reported in **millimeters of mercury.** In general, the International System of Units (SI) should be deferred to, although for some physiological measurements, other units have such widespread acceptance that SI units may seem a bit forced. Appropriate statistical methods are to be employed and described in detail, if they are not widely known.

With regard to clinical studies, CONSORT was the first set of guidelines to receive widespread acceptance and served as a model for others. An important feature of the CONSORT guidelines for methods sections is the emphasis on accounting for bias in the selection of subjects. This principle can be applied to the selection of cells or animals in basic scientific research or the selection of papers for inclusion in a systematic review. Journals also have their own reporting requirements for basic scientific studies, often based on academic societies' guidelines. These will require information which addresses the key issues of safety, humane treatment of animals, and the degree to which the experimental system approaches natural systems (i.e., validity).

Hence, guidelines tell us what to say, but what they seldom tell us is how to say it. How do effective writers actually present all of this information?

A useful general rule is that the methods section ought to describe the actual sequence of procedures as they were executed (13, 14). If our methodology is complex or the paper reports a number of different but related studies, this may not be possible. However, to the greatest extent possible, we should write our methods section as if it were to serve as instructions, much like a cook book, for other investigators. Clarity is sometimes served by dividing our methods section with sub-headings, and different journals often have their own guidelines in this regard. If we do use sub-headings for the methods section, these same sub-headings may also be used in the results section, and thereby improve the readability of the paper.

In practice, across genre, and even prior to the recent emergence of content guidelines, successful writers have characteristically incorporated into their methods sections three "moves" which parallel the recommendations of the Uniform Requirements. These moves are (i) identifying the source of data and the method adopted in collecting them; (ii) describing the experimental procedures and methods adopted in the processing of data and (iii) describing the procedures adopted in the analysis, including statistical analysis, of data (3). In writing our own methods section, we would be wise to follow this pattern, and fit our content to the sequence of moves.

Move 1 of the methods section identifies the nature and source of the cells, animals or people we are studying, for example "**Experiments were performed on 8 urethane-anesthetized adult male Wistar rats aged 8 to 12 weeks and weighing 360 to 430 g.**" In basic scientific studies, it is not unusual to name the company, laboratory or colleague who provided the cells, animals or other materials. In clinical studies, we define the demographic characteristics of our subjects, as in the following example: "**34 patients (16 females and 18 males) aged 24 to 32 years (mean 28 ± 2years) were recruited into a randomized, crossover trial of …**" If the subjects belonged to a particular group, rather than being recruited from the population at large, the defining features of the group should be specified. For example, we might say "**Subjects were recruited from among the student population of …**" or "**Subjects were recruited from patients who visited the outpatient facility …**"

In as much as we are reporting work previously performed, it is the normal practice to use the past tense throughout the methods section, as demonstrated in the examples above. Also, note the preference for the passive voice: "**patients … were recruited**" not "**we recruited patients**". Frequent use of the passive voice is conventional in the methods section.

In the past, authors might have separately listed the inclusion and exclusion criteria for human subjects. According to the most recent version of the Uniform Requirements, this is not required and many authors find it convenient to bundle inclusion and exclusion criteria into a single statement.

In Move 2 of the methods section, we introduce the actual experimental methods including gathering and processing of data. This move therefore represents the main substance of the methods section. Experimental steps are presented sequentially with generous use of temporal adverbials to orient the reader in time. For example, we may have sentences such as "**Next**, sections were incubated **for 1 hour** at 4°C in phosphate buffer …" Despite the "cook book" nature of this section, authors almost invariably avoid an outright listing of steps, but rather use conjuncts to construct a more reader-friendly narrative of the experimental protocol.

Where we are employing methods developed by others, we will want to cite the original papers. This will help us to economize on our writing, since we will not need to repeat in detail each step of the methodology. Hence, we often see sentences such as "**Specimens were prepared for histological examination as described previously** (3)**.**" Of course, any modifications of the cited methodology will need to be detailed and justified. However, in general, the methods section of a paper will have few (and perhaps no) citations.

As methods in different subspecialties of biomedicine are quite distinct, so is the vocabulary of respective papers. In particular, the nouns (substances and devices) and verbs are likely to be quite different in, for example, molecular biology versus pathology. Nonetheless, certain methods verbs crop up frequently across the genres (15). These are: analyse, apply, assess, carry out, collect, determine, evaluate, examine, follow, measure, observe, obtain, perform, receive, study, take, treat, use.

Interestingly, "**treat**" is more common in reference to cells and animals rather than individual people (15). Consequently, for whatever reason, authors are likely to say "The mice **were treated** with…" but, "The patients **received treatment**." General procedural verbs, such as "**perform**" and "**carry out**" are often used early in the methods section, even in Move 1, to introduce the experimental protocol (15). "**Collect**," "**obtain**" and "**take**" are used in the context of gathering specimens, for example "Blood samples **were obtained** on days 1, 5 and 7 of the study." As in Move 1 of the methods section, in Move 2 the past tense and passive voice predominate (3), and the tense of main verbs seldom changes within one paragraph.

Move 3 details the analysis of data, and so is not present in those observational papers which rely purely on raw data. As there is a mathematical character to this move, authors often pause to define (or refine) key variables. Thus, we have sentences such as "In this study, the neonatal period **was defined as** the period from …"

Where statistical analysis is used, tests are named and criteria for significance are usually stated. For example, we might see "Pretreatment and post-treatment **data were compared via the paired t-test**, when data were distributed normally, and **via the Wilcoxon signed rank test**, when data were not distributed normally. A **p value of .05** was used as the threshold for **statistical significance**."

The three moves of the methods section thus take us from the introduction of the source of our data – cells, animals or humans – to the processed data which will be presented in the results section of our paper.

Key Points

1. The methods section provides sufficient detail that a knowledgeable researcher could duplicate the study and a knowledgeable reader could judge internal and external validity.
2. This is normally accomplished in three "moves" in the following sequence:
    - Identifying the source of data and the method adopted in collecting them
    - Describing the experimental procedures and methods adopted in the processing of data
    - Describing the procedures adopted in the analysis (including statistical analysis) of data

7   The Passive Voice and I

One of the fundamental rules of English composition is that the important words should come at the beginning of the sentence. Rarely, we will save up an important word until the very end of the sentence, and this can have quite a dramatic affect. However, this kind of device can only be used sparingly or it looses its impact. Biomedical writing follows the convention of general English, and so at the very beginning of the sentence we usually get a clear signal of what the sentence is about. Thus, many (but not all) sentences can be written in one of two ways. Consider the following two examples:

1. **We incubated the slides overnight at room temperature in a polyclonal rabbit anti-rat erythrocyte antibody.**
2. **The slides were incubated by us overnight at room temperature in a polyclonal rabbit anti-rat erythrocyte antibody.**

Both sentences are grammatically correct and provide the same information. However, in the first sentence the word "we" is the subject. In the second sentence, "**slides**" is the subject and the researchers, represented as "**us**", become what is called the agent. In fact, the passive voice usually takes precisely this format:

subject + auxiliary verb + main verb (ed) + by + agent

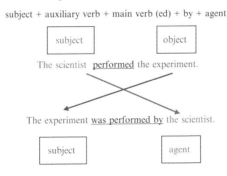

Sentence 1 expresses the action "**incubated**" in the active voice, but in sentence 2 the verb explodes into three words, "**were incubated by**". According to convention, the topic of sentence 1 is the researchers – "**we**", while sentence 2 is about "**the slides**". Which construction do you think better represents the intention of the authors?

Usually the active voice is thought to provide a more direct expression, and is a shorter sentence. Therefore, it is the preferred form in speaking and general writing. In fact, about 99% of general English sentences are written in the active voice. In scientific writing, however, the passive voice is quite common. For example, the passive voice accounts for about 33% of sentences in the nursing literature, 36% of sentences in the infectious diseases literature and more than 50% of sentences in the public health literature. The passive voice is especially common in the methods sections of papers and can make up more than 60% of main verbs (10). This proportion is so vastly different from general English that there must be a good reason for this convention.

Sentence 2 above will serve as a good example to explain the appeal of the passive voice. We have written it as:

"**The slides were incubated by us overnight at room temperature in a polyclonal rabbit anti-rat erythrocyte antibody.**"

In fact, this is somewhat contrived. The actual published sentence read:

"**The slides were incubated overnight at room temperature in a polyclonal rabbit anti-rat erythrocyte antibody.**"

The agent "**by us**" was eliminated in the published sentence. Therefore, the sentence was as short and readable as if it had been written in the active voice. This elimination of the agent happens in more than 80% of passive sentences in the biomedical literature, as in the following examples:

- Patients with mild to severe COPD **were recruited** from the respiratory department.
- Adult hemodialysis patients **were selected** using a computer generated list.
- This case-control study **was conducted** in Kyoto University Hospital.
- The patients with tube feeding **were randomized** to receive one of two regimes.
- Newborn information **was obtained** from birth records.

Hence, the argument that the active voice is more direct and readable does not hold up in practice. In research reports, and especially in the methods section, scientists report their own work. Including self reference – "**we**" – as the subject of an active voice sentence, or "**by us**" as the agent in a passive voice sentence is unnecessary and would be burdensome to the reader.

Additionally, in biomedical writing authors frequently begin their sentences with a word or phrase which announces the theme of the sentence. In the methods section, this word or phrase is most often the actual focus of the research – the cell, the rat or the patient, or a procedure – the selection, the treatment, the analysis (16). The sentences below illustrate this point:

- **Quality of life** was measured by …
- **Head injury** was defined by …

In each instance, the theme of the sentence is absolutely clear from the outset. Hence, the passive voice gives better service than the active voice on two counts. First, the construction of the passive voice places the focus of research activity at the beginning of the sentence and unmistakably announces the theme. Secondly, unnecessary self-reference by the author is avoided.

In fact, referring to ourselves directly – using "**I**" or "**We**" – is quite unusual and may even be considered bad form in the hard sciences (17). In other fields, writers may trade on their fame to establish claims, and so reference to themselves may render an argument more credible. However, in the biomedical arena, taking the personality out of our writing actually makes our manuscript more engaging and convincing to our readership (17). Thus, the pronoun "I" is virtually absent from biomedical papers, and "we" makes only a rare appearance in the methods section when it is necessary to accentuate some distinctive feature of our protocol (18).

The convention of impersonality is so strong in the biomedical literature that when we cannot find a passive sentence construction which fits our needs, we may go to what might be called "pseudo-passive" devices (18). For example, rather than "**The researchers gave treatment to the patients …**" we will see "**The patients received treatment …**". The verb "**received**" is in the active voice, but achieves the important task of rendering the researchers invisible. Here are some other examples using this popular verb:

- They **received** ambulatory oxygen ...
- ...randomized **to receive** either half-solid enteral nutriments ...
- Those who **received** care for chronic neurologic sequelae were not included.

Similarly, "**Vaccination resulted in the development of immunity in** ..." deliberately eliminates reference to whoever performed the act of vaccination. It is not uncommon to find such instances where inanimate objects or abstractions are almost given human-like volition.

Hence, various devices are used by successful authors to draw attention away from themselves and towards the act of research. This is a striking feature of biomedical writing and apparently serves an important role in establishing a relationship of trust between writer and reader.

Key Points

1. The passive voice is used much more often in biomedical writing than in general English, and it is the most prevalent form of the main verb in the methods sections of papers.
2. This use of the passive voice is appropriate and effective in conveying meaning with clarity. In particular, it is a useful device in establishing the research act as the theme of sentences.
3. Where a passive construction is not convenient, writers may resort to "pseudo-passive" devices.
4. Reference to self is uncommon, and the pronoun "I" is almost absent from biomedical writing.
5. Collectively, these conventions render biomedical writing more engaging and convincing to a scientific readership.

8 Writing an Effective Results Section

The results section of our paper ought to be the easiest section to write, and actually this often turns out to be the case, especially if we have been true to the purpose of our study and have rigorously tested our research hypothesis.

The results section of the paper should also be the most objective section. It presents the unadorned data with a minimum amount of explanation. This allows the reader to form their own judgments about the meaning of the results. Certainly, if our study is exploratory, rather than challenging a dichotomous hypothesis, a modicum of interpretation may be useful to keep the reader on track. However, to the greatest extent possible, explanations and interpretations should be kept for the discussion section.

The Uniform Requirements tell us that we need to think of the most logical sequence in which to present our data, and this is often (but not invariably) the sequence in which results were actually obtained in our study. Since the results are the informative core of the paper, this section needs to set out our observations in adequate detail and in a form which facilitates interpretation. Content guidelines, such as CONSORT and STARD, are quite clear about the information which ought to be included in manuscripts. However, detailed genre-specific guidelines for basic scientific studies have yet to emerge, and in part this might be due to an assumption that the contents of the results section ought to be obvious. In practice, however, this assumption is not always correct. Increasingly, basic scientific studies are relying upon the processing of information, so that there is a tendency to omit raw data for economy's sake. Better journals, however, will insist on seeing at least representative examples of raw data – the real results – and will want to see how computed values are derived from these data (with the appropriate number of significant figures).

We may want to present more than one analysis of our data, even if the interpretations of these analyses are inconsistent in some way. While one might be inclined to think that this would undermine a paper, in fact it tends to engage readers by inviting them to consider the data for themselves and settle on their own conclusions. Even so, we will want to be clear about which analyses were planned and which were post hoc.

It is often useful to present data in tables or figures. However, we need to be conservative. Tables with too much data are difficult to comprehend, and such data may be better served by a graph. Furthermore, we should not use tables and graphs when it is possible to present the same data with clarity within the text of the paper.

The items comprising the contents of the results section therefore seem easy enough to determine. Furthermore, not only is the content straightforward, but also the style used by successful writers is quite simple and direct. Normally, the results section consists of only one or two "moves". The ubiquitous move is the presentation of observations which were consistent with our expectations or hypothesis. Additionally, some papers include a second move which presents our inconsistent observations (3).

The first move of the results section often has an introductory statement which summarizes the observations or orients the reader to the text to follow; for example "**The clinical outcomes at 1, 3 and 6 months are presented below.**" This is then followed by characteristic cycles, each composed of three steps (19). The three steps are:

1. A metatextual expression referring to later text or a visual element; e.g. "**Mean blood pressures for the two groups are shown in fig. 1.**"
2. A statement of the results; e.g. "**The treatment group had lower mean arterial pressure than the control group.**"
3. A substantiation or reiteration of the results; e.g. "**At 3 months, MAP in the treatment group was 10 ± 3 mmHg lower than in the control group ($p \leq 0.01$).**"

Step one is directing the readers' attention to text which exists below or to data which exists in an accompanying illustration or table. Hence, the constituent sentences are written in the present tense. The active and passive voice are used with approximately the same frequency. Thus, we might see either, "**The data are shown in figure 2**" or "**Figure 2 shows the data.**"

Step 2 is the actual statement of results obtained when the research was performed, and so is almost invariably written in the past tense. The passive voice is conventional in this element of the results. Whereas step 1 is achieved in a single sentence, or even in a single phrase, step 2 is more substantial and makes up more than three quarters of the text in results sections.

Step 3 is also characterized by the past tense and the passive voice. It may contain details to substantiate step 2. There may also be evaluative expressions which perhaps are intended to encourage certain interpretations of the data, for example "**As expected**, blood pressure dropped following administration of propranolol" begs the question of who was doing the expecting (and whether readers are allowed to expect other outcomes).

The cycle of three steps is repeated as the authors work through all of their data. In basic scientific papers, the progression of cycles usually follows the chronology of the methods. In a physiological study for example, cycles might trace an animal's heart rate or blood pressure over a period of hours and in response to various stimuli. In epidemiological and clinical studies, on the other hand, the successive cycles may deal with different cohorts who actually went through the investigation concurrently. For example, the first cycle may deal with outcomes for patients who had certain risk factors. Then the second cycle might deal with patients who did not have those risk factors.

The flow from one cycle to the next may be facilitated by conjunctive expressions such as "**On the other hand**, at follow up the advantage of combined therapy was not so evident." Cycles may also be introduced by procedural phrases or sentences which serve to remind the reader of the methods; for example "In the second group, **which commenced rehabilitation on day 2 following surgery**, recovery of function was significantly better." Such procedural sentences frequently make use of the verbs "**perform**", "**assess**", "**apply**" and "**investigate**", and characteristically use the passive voice (19). We also occasionally encounter sentences describing modifications of procedures, especially in physiological papers, and CONSORT actually specifies that we should describe an deviations from our planned protocol in clinical trials.

Move 2, when present, is likely to follow the same steps as Move 1, but is more abbreviated. Although "negative" results (results not consistent with our expectations or hypothesis) may be important to our understanding of clinical or basic scientific issues, they make rather flat reading and cannot constitute a substantial portion of the results section. Even when such observations do not represent an experimental failure, it is hard to escape the implication that if our original research plan had been better thought out, our observations would have been a better match for our expectations.

Key Points

1. The results section presents the unadorned data with a minimum of discussion.
2. The results section invariably contains a move which presents those data which were consistent with the research hypothesis or our expectations. Additionally, there may be a second move which discusses results which were not consistent with the hypothesis or expectations.
3. Normally, a move contains cycles of three steps: (i) referring to the data (often in an accompanying figure); (ii) stating the results and (iii) substantiating or reiterating the results.

9   The Special Case of Case Studies

Case studies are retrospective studies in which observations were made in the course of interventions. Hence, the IMRAD format of experimental studies is not appropriate. In case studies, we make certain observations (what we would normally think of as "results") and then we provide some intervention, which we are inclined to think of as "methods". In case studies, these two portions of the report are presented in sections which may be termed "Case Presentation" and "Management and Outcome."

In the Case Presentation, we first describe the complaint that brought the patient to us. For example, we often see sentences such as "**A 45 year old mother of 2 presented with recurrent right upper quadrant abdominal pain.**" The pattern of "[patient] … **presented with** … [complaint]" may seem a bit hackneyed, but it is an efficient and comprehensible way to introduce the case.

Next, we introduce the important information that we obtained from our history-taking. It is often helpful to use the patient's own words. We don't need to include every detail – just the information that helped us to settle on our diagnosis. Also, we should try to present patient information in a narrative form – full sentences which efficiently summarize the results of our questioning. In our own clinical practices, the history usually leads to a differential diagnosis – a short list of the most likely diseases or disorders underlying the patient's symptoms. We may or may not choose to include this list at the end of this section of the case presentation.

The next step is to describe the results of our clinical examination. Again, we should write in an efficient narrative style, restricting ourselves to the relevant information. For example, if the patient came in suffering from an acute whiplash injury we probably don't need to be told that their temperature was normal, and we certainly don't need to be told that it was 37°C. That is not to say that we shouldn't be taking patients' temperatures in our practices – it simply means that such information does not help the case report.

If we are using a named test, for example the "**Jackson test**", it is best to both name and describe the test (since some people may know the test by a different name). Also, we should describe the actual results, since there may be some confusion about what constitutes a "**positive**"or "**negative**" result. Similarly, if we are presenting laboratory results, it is useful to provide the lab's normal values, since these may vary.

Based on the history and examination of the patient, we will have arrived at an assessment/diagnosis which is the basis for our management plan. In the "Management and Outcome" section of our paper, we set out clearly the plan for care, the care which was actually provided, and the outcome.

In describing our management, it is important for the reader to know how long the patient was under care (how many weeks or months) and how many times they were treated. Additionally, we should be as specific as possible in describing the treatment that we used. It does not help the reader to simply say that the patient received physical therapy. Specifically, what modalities did we use?

The patient's reports of improvement (or worsening) are useful. However, whenever possible we should try to use a well-validated method of measuring their improvement. For example, we might use data from visual analogue scales (VAS) for pain, or a journal of medication usage. If this information can be summarized in a table, or better yet a chart, it is more easily absorbed by the reader.

This portion of our case study might conclude with an indication of how and why treatment finished. Did we discharge the patient, and if so, why? Did the patient decide to terminate care? Did we refer the patient to another practitioner.

Case reports are often written by field practitioners with no experience in experimental research. They are frequently novice writers who may be inclined to use scientific jargon or include excessive detail, perhaps feeling that this will add credibility. Case reports, however, are founded on trust between colleagues – by their nature they document irreproducible events. It is their unpretentious manner and leanness of writing which engage readers.

Key Points

1. Reporting of case studies or case series normally does not follow the IMRAD format.
2. The value of case studies lays within the details concerning the individual patients and interventions, but unnecessary detail and scientific jargon will not engage readers.

10 Writing an Effective Discussion

The discussion may be the most challenging part of the paper to write, since we have to make sense of results which are seldom exactly as anticipated. Many papers fall apart in the discussion as writers struggle to find clarity in their results. It is at this point that the wisdom of a dichotomous (yes or no) hypothesis becomes obvious.

In order to avoid difficulty, the discussion should focus on the results of the current study and not extrapolate too broadly. Individual studies tend to make incremental advances in knowledge, and it is understood that questions will remain to be answered by future studies. On the other hand, an effort must be made to relate the findings of the current work to established knowledge and current theories. This is where the average reader looks for value – in the synthesis of new information to create a broader understanding of a particular area of science.

In general, the discussion section therefore consists of three moves (3). These are:
1. Highlighting the Overall Research Outcome
2. Explaining Specific Research Outcomes
3. Stating Research Conclusions

Move 1 of the discussion is often an explicit affirmation that the researchers performed the experiments that they set out to perform, or answered their research question. The move may consist of a single sentence following this sort of model:

"This study investigated the effect of … on …"

or

"This study investigated the effectiveness of … in [verb] + ing"

For example, we may see "**This study investigated the effect of a community-based educational program on quality of life among patients suffering from Parkinsonism.**" There does not need to be reference to the actual results – in this case, whether or not the intervention was successful – simply that the study was completed.

Move 2 of the discussion is much more extensive, reviewing and explaining the results in detail. This is achieved in a number of steps as follows:

(i) A reiteration of the main observations; e.g. "**This study found that** a community-based educational program improved the quality of life of patients with Parkinsonism." As the study has been completed, the statement is characteristically in the past tense. Alternatively, we may find statements such as "**These findings suggest that** a community-based educational program can improve the quality of life of patients with Parkinsonism." As the findings persist after completion of the study, this example uses the present tense. Both of our examples use the structure [verb] + *that* …

(ii) The second step in Move 2 is an explicit statement of the significance of the results; for example "**The importance of these findings is that …**" or "**A significant outcome of this study is that…**" Both of these examples are written in the present tense as is characteristic of this step.

(iii) The third step justifies the results by confirming that the methods were appropriate to the research question. For example, we see sentences such as "Permanent implantation of electrodes **was thus necessary** to achieve reproducible recordings in our study."

(iv) The fourth step compares and contrasts our new results with those of previous studies. This section is often introduced with a very explicit signal that we are juxtaposing our results against those of others. For example, we may say "**Our findings are similar to** those of Tanaka et al., who observed that …" or "**The present study differs from** previous studies in including…" This comparison is a crucial step in demonstrating how our study contributes to the common body of knowledge. It essentially justifies the performance of the research (and publication of the paper), and may represent a particularly vulnerable point for clinical studies (20).

(v) The fifth and final step in Move 2 discusses the limitations in our paper and in those we have cited, including technical limitations imposed by the methods (for example the accuracy of diagnostic tests used in the study) and limitations on interpretation, including external validity. Sentences may begin with explicit preparatory phrases: "**Some limitations of the current study are** the relatively small sample size and …"

Move 3 states our conclusions. This is done quite explicitly and is frequently signaled by the use of words such as "**conclusion**" and "**summary**". For example:

"**In summary**, the spinal cord undergoes viscoelastic relaxation during sustained compression."
"**In conclusion**, the significance of this study is that …"

This move most often provides the "yes or no" answer to our hypothesis, or makes the definitive statement about what the study has achieved. There is likely to be a statement of research questions which arise from this study, and therefore suggestions for further research, for example "**What needs to be investigated further is** whether or not …"

In clinical papers, there will be a statement of the implications for patient care. For example, we may suggest "The measures used in our study **may help to identify treatment methods** that…"

Key Points

1. The discussion consists of three moves: (i) Highlighting the Overall Research Outcome, (ii) Explaining Specific Research Outcomes and (iii) Stating Research Conclusions.
2. An essential function of the discussion is to place the results of the current study within the context of current knowledge. This step is critical in justifying the study and justifying publication of the paper.

11 Is It a Discussion or a Systematic Review?

Less experienced writers often find that too much of their discussion seems to be duplicating what they have already written. It is, in fact, a real challenge to place our own results in context without simply recycling the introduction (and methods and results). There are, of course, important parallels between the introduction and discussion, but there are also clear differences in discourse and style.

The introduction describes our understanding of the field when we commenced our research (21) and proceeds from this broad perspective to the small niche which we wish to claim. The discussion proceeds in the opposite direction from our relatively small contribution to broader implications (11). Not surprisingly, therefore, the discussion is the most heavily hedged section of our paper, making generous use of shields (especially modal verbs) and compound hedges, e.g. "**These results seem to suggest that …**" or "**It appears reasonable to assume that …**"

Of course, we may need to discuss certain key references from the introduction and refer to certain details of our protocols and data, but we do not reiterate these sections at length. Furthermore, whereas the methods and results sections were essentially factual renditions of what was done and what happened, the discussion is argumentative (in the literary sense). This is where we try to persuade the reader. This very clear transition in styles is reflected in the themes of our sentences. In the methods and results sections of our paper, the subjects of our sentences are the objects and procedures of research: patients, rats, cells and proteins; treatment, diagnosis, microscopy and so forth. In the discussion section, the themes of our sentences are largely abstractions reflecting thought processes – not what we did or whom we did it to, but what we think about all of that (16). Commonly occurring themes of sentences are so called "epistemic nouns" including:

analysis(es), assumption, difference, distribution, evidence, finding, increase, levels, method, model, nature, observation, probabilities, proportion, rate, response, result(s), study(ies), variation, work.

The persuasive nature of this section is also signaled by the frequent use of adversative conjuncts such as "**however**" and "**nevertheless**". Authors also try to influence readers with adverbials including "**indeed**", "**interestingly**", "**(un)fortunately**" and "**importantly**".

Hence, the discussion is the persuasive counterpoint to the factual and quantitative methods and results sections of our paper.

Content guidelines such as CONSORT and STARD ask that we place our study in context and offer clinical implications. It has even been suggested that, for clinical papers, the discussion should include a systematic review incorporating the current results (20). In practice, however, this ideal has not achieved support in clinical or basic scientific writing. The discussion remains the persuasive, not the quantitative, heart of the paper.

Key Points

1. In terms of pattern of discourse and style, the discussion is quite different from the introduction. The introduction proceeds from a broad perspective to a narrow focus, whereas the discussion proceeds from restricted findings to broad implications.
2. The methods and results sections of papers are quantitative, whereas the discussion is the persuasive core of the paper, as is reflected in the themes of sentences and the choices of verbs.
3. In practice, the discussion does not present an extensive review of the literature, as this would be redundant of the introduction.

12 Writing an Effective Abstract

An abstract is a very concise overview of a study, usually appended to the beginning of the full report. Although the abstract characteristically appears at the beginning of the paper, it is often (and probably ought to be) the last thing that we write. Like the title, the composition of the abstract should be undertaken thoughtfully with the view of winning over editors, reviewers and readers.

There are two broad divisions of abstract: narrative and structured. In the past, abstracts often took the form of a narrative: a continuous series of sentences which described the study from start to finish. While a narrative is perhaps easier to read, a lack of formal structure may mean that certain important information is excluded. Hence, there is now a strong trend towards structured abstracts: abstracts with subdivisions each accorded certain content.

This movement is fueled by the need of research consumers to search large libraries of articles in order to find the material which suits their particular requirements. Often, decisions about which articles to download and read are based on the contents of the abstract. Especially as electronic search engines are more often used to identify articles of interest, the content of abstracts becomes critical to improving access to relevant articles.

Concerning the content of abstracts, the Uniform Requirements have this to say:

> The abstract should provide the context or background for the study and should state the study's purposes, basic procedures (selection of study subjects or laboratory animals, observational and analytical methods), main findings (giving specific effect sizes and their statistical significance, if possible), and principal conclusions. It should emphasize new and important aspects of the study or observations.

These days, the majority of articles in high-impact journals use structured abstracts, and more than two thirds of these use the **introduction, methods, results** and **discussion** (IMRAD) format. It is often possible to copy and paste summary sentences from the text of the article for the introduction and discussion portions of the abstract. The methods and results portions of the abstract will require some distillation of the corresponding sections of the study.

The other popular format for abstracts of clinical studies uses eight-points: **objective, design, setting, patients, interventions, main outcome measures, results** and **conclusions.** It is not uncommon to see these sections written in point form rather than in full sentences (see the examples below) and the relevant information is stated very explicitly. Interestingly, the conclusions are often written in the present tense and active voice to emphasize their generalizability and the confidence of the author. This is in contrast to the more circumspect writing found in the main text.

Examples

Objective

i. We sought to determine the optimal dose of the selective endothelin A (ET(A)) receptor antagonist sitaxsentan for the treatment of pulmonary arterial hypertension (PAH).
ii. Our objective was to determine the incidence of and patient/treatment factors associated with AOF in a large cohort of pediatric cancer survivors.
iii. To determine the effects of CEE on breast cancers and mammographic findings.

Design

i. We conducted a retrospective cohort, multicenter study.
ii. In this double-blind, placebo-controlled 18-week study, 247 PAH patients (idiopathic, or associated with connective tissue disease or congenital heart disease) were randomized.
iii. Prospective, double blind, randomised, placebo controlled trial.

Setting

i. The Alfred Hospital, Melbourne, Australia
ii. Primary care, among a randomly selected group of general practitioners in Christchurch, New Zealand
iii. University hospital

Patients

i. Forty older adults with symptomatic PAD and no history of diabetes or hypertension.
ii. Fifty-nine women aged 16–50 years presenting with a history of dysuria and frequency in whom a dipstick test of midstream urine was negative for both nitrites and leucocytes. Participants with complicated urinary tract infection were excluded.
iii. Thirty patients on cardiopulmonary bypass undergoing coronary artery bypass grafting.

Interventions

i. Ten milligrams of ramipril (n = 20) or placebo (n = 20) once daily for 24 weeks. All patients completed the trial.
ii. A dose of 0.625 mg/day of CEE or an identical-appearing placebo.
iii. Patients received 5,000 units/kg intravenous urinary trypsin inhibitor (n = 15) or 0.9% saline (control, n = 15) immediately before aortic cannulation for cardiopulmonary bypass.

Main Outcome Measures

i. The primary end point was change in 6 MW distance from baseline to week 18. Secondary end points included change in WHO FC, time to clinical worsening, and change in Borg dyspnea score.
ii. Pain-free and maximum walking time were recorded during a standard treadmill test, and the standard Walking Impairment Questionnaire was administered.
iii. Breast cancer incidence, tumor characteristics, and mammogram findings.

Results

i. Regular non-aspirin and any NSAID use increased from 0% to 12% and 1% to 56% over time, respectively and was predicted by age, body mass index, alcohol consumption, medication use, coronary artery disease, gastrointestinal diseases, arthritis, hypertension, and headaches.

ii. At week 18, patients treated with sitaxsentan 100 mg had an increased 6MW distance compared with the placebo group (31.4 m, p = 0.03), and an improved WHO FC (p = 0.04).

iii. After adjustment for the baseline pain-free walking time, mean pain-free walking time after ramipril treatment was 227 s (95% CI, 175 s to 278 s; p < 0.001) longer than that after placebo treatment.

Conclusions

i. Treatment with the selective ET(A) receptor antagonist sitaxsentan, orally once daily at a dose of 100 mg, improves exercise capacity and WHO FC in PAH patients, with a low incidence of hepatic toxicity.

ii. Ramipril improved pain-free and maximum walking time in some adults with symptomatic PAD.

iii. HF risk decreased with chlorthalidone versus amlodipine or lisinopril use during year 1.

For review articles, a six-point format is also used: **purpose, data sources, study selection, data extraction, results of data synthesis and conclusions.** As review articles attempt to synthesize from many studies, the conclusions section of the abstract tends to be more hedged that in basic scientific and clinical studies.

Abstracts of case studies and case series often follow a different format:
Introduction: consisting of one or two sentences to summarize the entire article.
Case presentation: describing the history and results of any examinations performed. The processes of diagnosis and management are also described in this section.
Outcome: A straightforward record of the course of the patient's complaint. Where possible, reference is made to any outcome measures that were used

to objectively demonstrate how the patient's condition evolved through the course of management.

Conclusions: A brief assessment of the lessons learned from the case.

Structured abstracts obviously work best for well structured research, such as basic scientific studies, prospective clinical trials, structured reviews and meta-analyses. Well accepted formats have yet to emerge for abstracts of observational and qualitative studies.

Abstracts are intended to provide, economically and objectively, the main points of the article. Nonetheless, authors may insinuate evaluative expressions as part of the process of persuading readers of the value of their article (22). These persuasive devices include

Modifiers of verbs

e.g. "**Interestingly, these results point to ...**"

Evaluative nouns

e.g. "**The importance/relevance of these findings is ...**"

Modality, especially within the background and conclusions sections

e.g. "**These results suggest that ...**"

Modal verbs occur somewhat less frequently in the abstract that in other portions of the report, and the passive voice is decidedly less common in the abstract (10). This may reflect the need for economy in abstracts, which often have stringent limits on word count. This relative lack of hedging may also signal the desire of authors to make strong assertions in order to gain the attention of potential readers.

Key Points

1. The abstract provides an important opportunity to win over editors, reviewers and readers. This section of the paper deserves as much

thoughtful composition as any other section as it will often be the deciding factor in whether or not a paper is published or read.
2. Abstracts tend to be more direct and confident in their statements than other portions of the paper.

13 The Process of Manuscript Submission and Review

Especially for novice writers, the process of composing a manuscript can be quite exhausting. When we have finally completed our paper, it is, in our minds, as good as we can make it and we are justifiably proud and relieved. However, we must also realize that what we have in our hands is an unpublished manuscript. All of our work is wasted unless we can convince a journal to publish our paper. Therefore it is important to maintain our focus and give full attention to the processes involved in shepherding our paper through submission and review to successful publication.

Fortunately, there are no mysteries to the process of paper submission. The Uniform Requirements contain detailed instructions on the preparation of manuscripts, and these guidelines, with perhaps some minor amendments, have been adopted by the overwhelming majority of biomedical journals. In fact, the Uniform Requirements may actually contain more detail that we need; for example instructions on the order in which to layout text, references, tables and figures. This excess of detail arises because the Uniform Requirements were developed for an age when manuscripts were still submitted in paper form. These days, almost all journals accept electronic submissions and many make electronic submission mandatory. Not only does this speed up the review process, but it means that much of the detail of submission can be left up to the computer. For these reasons, it is a good idea early in the process of writing to check with the journal web site and see how they can assist with submission.

These days, submitting a paper normally means going to the journal's home page and logging on through an area for authors. The author is asked to register and obtain a user identification and password. This is best done well in advance of submission, since it permits us to become familiar with our target journal's processes and this can save us a lot of work later. Also, the process of registering as an author can be somewhat time-consuming and we may not have the energy to do this and submit our manuscript all in one session.

Once we begin the process of manuscript submission, we do not need to complete it all at once. We can log on and off as often as necessary, submitting individual sections of our paper as they are completed. We can also withdraw previously submitted files and substitute new ones as necessary. In many instances, we can copy the text from our own files and paste it into a template on the journal web site. The journal's system will then automatically convert the text to the appropriate font and size, indenting and spacing according to their style and so saving us a great deal of work. When all of this is done and we are completely satisfied with our paper, we are then able to submit it for review. In practice this usually means informing the system that we are ready to submit, at which point the system will generate a draft, usually in pdf format. This gives us a final chance to see the manuscript in exactly the form that the editor and reviewers will see it. Almost invariably, we will find some minor typographical errors or awkward phraseology that we will choose to correct. Then we approve the submission and off it goes to the editor for review.

The process of review may seem an opaque and stressful experience for authors as the fate of their manuscript is decided by often-anonymous reviewers. However, a familiarity with the normal events of review can make the whole process easier to navigate. The actual steps will be determined by each journal. With small journals the entire process may fall to a single editor and a handful of reviewers operating in rather an *ad hoc* manner. Higher-impact journals will have stricter standard operating procedures administered by a hierarchy of editorial staff.

In the past, submitted manuscripts may have taken months to review, and during that time the author had no sense of what had become of their work. These days it is often possible to track the progress of a submission through the journal's web site, and so there is less mystery involved. Also, the entire process generally proceeds more efficiently these days. At the larger journals, submitted manuscripts are received and screened by a handling editor who may make a preliminary judgement based only on reading the abstract. In this way, the handling editor may make a quick decision not to accept articles which are not sufficiently original, interesting or central to the scope of the journal. It may seem severe to the author to have laboured months on a manuscript and then have it rejected within days or even hours of submission. However, it also means that the authors can quickly submit their manuscript to a more appropriate journal without having to wait months (during which time their research may become dated). If the article survives that first screening, the handling editor will likely read the entire manuscript and again make a judgement on suitability for the journal. They may also recognize important scientific errors which make a paper unacceptable.

If our manuscript survives this process, it will be sent out for external review, usually by two or three reviewers with expertise in the area of the paper. At the better journals, about 2/3 s of submissions have already been eliminated by this point.

Reviewers are unpaid and busy colleagues who nonetheless volunteer their efforts in order to assist journals. When they and the authors have both done their jobs, a good paper is improved and everyone benefits. However, reviewers are generally in short supply, and journals struggle to find qualified experts. For this reason, you may be asked to nominate your own reviewers. This has benefits for all. Author-nominated reviewers are often experts in the field, and provide reviews of good quality – comparable to those of reviewers nominated by the journal (23). On the other hand, and not surprisingly, they are generally more sympathetic in their recommendations about acceptance of a submission. For these reasons, if a journal gives us the opportunity to nominate our own reviewers, we should definitely take advantage of this option.

Historically, authors have been blinded to the identity of reviewers and reviewers have generally not been told the identity of authors. This seems like a system which would facilitate fairness. It protects reviewers from intimidation, just as it shield authors who may have produced a less than perfect first draft. There is also clear evidence that knowledge of author identity or affiliation influences the judgement of reviewers (24). Thus, blinding seems like a good idea, but in fact has mixed success. The truth is that reviewers, being familiar with who is doing what within their field, can often guess the identities of authors so that anonymity is one-sided (25). This clearly places authors at a disadvantage. Thus, more recently a number of journals have moved towards open review in which both authors and reviewers are identified. There is good evidence that such open review improves the quality of reviews and, happily for authors, results in more sympathetic recommendations.

Most often, reviewers will make recommendations for some revision of a manuscript. For many authors this is a very positive experience as they have the benefit of expert opinion which can save them from publishing flawed science or a poorly formulated paper. On the other hand, very severe criticisms will result in a paper being rejected or the authors being required to make major revisions. Only rarely is a paper accepted without any recommendations for revision. On the basis of the reviewers' comments, the editor(s) will then make a decision about the disposition of the paper.

Normally, when reviewers are recruited, they are asked to commit to completing their work within a period of time – perhaps 3 weeks. If they feel that they cannot satisfy this requirement, the editor will look for an alternative reviewer. All of this means that by the time two or three reviewers have been recruited and have completed their work, 6 or 8 weeks may have passed since submission. For anxious authors, this seems interminable, but the process is not finished yet.

Even a good, publishable paper may not be published if a journal is overwhelmed with high-quality submissions. This is the case with the better journals. Therefore editorial staff may discuss their acceptable papers and decide which are of highest merit. Of course, the scientific quality of a paper is very important. However, much consideration is also given to the importance of the findings and their relevance to the mission of the journal (26).

A significant challenge for all authors is knowing how to respond to reviewers' criticisms. Initially, it is hard not to take offence at some comments. After all, we have normally put a great deal of effort into our writing and have been hoping for a favourable reception. It is therefore important to take a dispassionate view of reviewers' comments and even attempt to find the positive aspects. Especially if two or three reviewers have identified the same weakness in our paper, we can be fairly certain that the fault is ours, not theirs. Furthermore, even if we conclude that a particular comment is overly harsh, the most efficient route to publication is to try to satisfy the reviewer. We do not want to be intimidated into publishing incorrect results or conclusions, but reviewers are in short supply, whereas many journals have an overabundance of aspiring authors. For this reason, editors would rather see revisions than rebuttals to reviewers' comments. If one truly wishes to argue some point, it is best to be well armed with referenced evidence.

For non-native English speakers, the quality of science may be less of an issue than the matter of constructing convincing arguments. In part, this has to do with concrete issues of spelling and grammar, but also involves conventions of discourse which may be influenced by socio-cultural sensitivities (6). In other words, the way in which something is normally expressed in our own language may be overly abrupt or obtuse when translated into English. Many editors make allowance for these differences, and it is not necessary to have native-like English fluency in order to be published, even in the better journals. Nonetheless, the better the English is, the more likely the paper is to be accepted. Particularly if a paper has been returned with comments on the language, these must be addressed as seriously as comments on scientific matters.

Key Points

1. Articles may be quickly rejected solely on the merit of the abstract and so authors need to put much effort into crafting an abstract which will appeal to their target journal.
2. If permitted, it is beneficial to the authors to nominate their own reviewers. This increases the likelihood of acceptance without undermining the quality of the review.
3. Rebuttals to reviewers' comments are less productive than compliant revisions.

Epilogue – Our Shared Biomedical Language

This book is about biomedical writing – the expression of the experience of our research culture through our **biomedical language**. Most of us who publish in biomedicine are not native English speakers, but it is we who have stewardship over our language. **Biomedical language** is sufficiently distinctive that it is largely incomprehensible to most native English speakers. Apart from an extensive and esoteric vocabulary, there are, as we have seen in the preceding chapters, particular conventions in grammar and discourse. All of us who wish to enjoy success in this unique language – whether we are native English speakers or not – need to undertake serious, enjoyable study of this rich medium. Knowledge of our shared **biomedical language** is an incredibly powerful tool for turning marginal biomedical writing into solid, convincing discourse. This book began with the assumption that we are all learners, but as stewards of the language, we also have the wonderful opportunity to invent and improve on our developing language.

References

1. Bredan A, van Roy F. Writing readable prose. EMBO Reports 2006;7(9):846–849.
2. Soler V. Writing titles in science: an exploratory study. English for Specific Purposes 2007;26:90–102.
3. Nwogu K. The medical research paper: structure and functions. English for Specific Purposes 1997;16(2):119–138.
4. Thomas S, Hawes T. Reporting verbs in medical journal articles. English for Specific Purposes 1994;13(2):129–148.

5. Salager-Meyer F, Angeles M, Ariza A, Zambrano N. The scimitar, the dagger and the glove: intercultural differences in the rhetoric of criticism in Spanish, French and English medical discourse (1930–1995). English for Specific Purposes 2003;22:223–247.
6. Gosden H. 'Why not give us the full story?': functions of referee's comments in peer reviews of scientific research papers. Journal of English for Academic Purposes 2003;2:87–101.
7. Lewin B. Hedging: an exploratory study of authors' and readers' identification of 'toning down' in scientific texts. Journal of English for Academic Purposes 2005;4:163–178.
8. Varttala T. Remarks on the communicative functions of hedging in popular scientific and specialist research articles on medicine. English for Specific Purposes 1999;18(2):177–200.
9. Smith D. Medical discourse: aspects of author's comment. The ESP Journal 1984;3:25–36.
10. Salager-Meyer F. A text-type and move analysis study of verb tense and modality distribution in medical English abstracts. English for Specific Purposes 1992;11:93–113.
11. Salager-Meyer F. Hedges and textual communicative function in medical English written discourse. English for Specific Purposes 1994;13(2):149–170.
12. Mungra P. A research and discussion note: the macrostructure of consensus statements. English for Specific Purposes 2007;26.
13. Kallet R. How to write the methods section of a research paper. Respiratory Care 2004;49(10):1229–1232.
14. Coverdale J. Writing the methods. Academic Psychiatry 2006;30(5):361–364.
15. Williams I. A contextual study of lexical verbs in two types of medical research report: clinical and experimental. English for Specific Purposes 1996;15(3):175–197.
16. Martinez I. Aspects of theme in the method and discussion sections of biology journal articles in English. Journal of English for Academic Purposes 2003;2:103–123.
17. Hyland K. Humble servants of the discipline? Self-mention in research articles. English for Specific Purposes 2001;20:207–226.
18. Martinez I. Impersonality in the research article as revealed by analysis of the transitivity structure. English for Specific Purposes 2001;20:227–247.
19. Williams I. Results sections of medical research articles: analysis of rhetorical categories for pedagogical purposes. English for Specific Purposes 1999;18(4):347–366.
20. Clarke M, Chalmers I. Discussion sections in reports of controlled trials published in general medical journals. Journal of the American Medical Association 1998;280(3):280–282.

21. Wells W. Unpleasant surprises: how the introduction has wandered into the discussion. The Journal of Cell Biology 2006;174(6):741.
22. Stotesbury H. Evaluation in research article abstracts in the narrative and hard sciences. Journal of English for Academic Purposes 2003;2:327–341.
23. Schroter S, Tite L, Hutchings A, Black N. Differences in review quality and recommendations for publication between peer reviewers suggested by authors or by editors. JAMA 2006;295:314–317.
24. Ross JS, Gross CP, Desai MM, Hong Y, Grant AO, Daniels SR, Hachinski VC, Gibbons RJ, Gardner TJ, Krumholz HM. Effect of blinded peer review on abstract acceptance. JAMA 2006;295:1675–1680.
25. Godlee F. Making reviewers visible – openness, accountability, and credit. JAMA 2002;287:2762–2765.
26. Dickersin K, Ssemanda E, Mansell C, Rennie D. What do the JAMA editors say when they discuss manuscripts that they are considering for publication? Developing a schema for classifying the content of editorial discussion. BMC Medical Research Methodology 2007;7:44.

Index

abbreviations 10
abstract 2, 10, 49–54, 57
acronyms 10
active voice 32, 33, 36, 50
adverbials 10, 21, 48
adverbials, locative 10
adverbials, temporal 10, 27
approximators 22

background (see also "context") 8, 10, 12, 49, 53
biomedical language 61
blinded review 57

case presentation 39, 51
case series 1, 9, 51, 52
case studies 1, 2, 9, 39–41, 52
citations (see also "references") 10, 11, 28
clinical studies 26, 27, 37, 45, 52
conclusions 36, 43, 45, 49, 50, 51, 52, 53
conjuncts 15–17, 28, 37, 48
conjuncts, contrastive 12, 17
conjuncts, inference 16
conjuncts, listing 16, 17
conjuncts, simile 16
conjuncts, summarizing 16, 17
conjuncts, transition 16

conjunctions 15–17
consensus statements 22, 23
CONSORT 3, 4, 9, 26, 35, 37, 48
content guidelines 3, 9, 26, 35, 48
context (see also "background") 9, 10, 13, 45, 46, 48, 49

design 2, 3, 9, 24, 50
differential diagnosis 39
discussion 2, 20, 21, 22, 23, 34, 38, 43–48, 50

epidemiological studies 37
exclusion criteria 27

figures 36

generalizability 25, 50
graphs 36

hedging 18, 19–23, 47, 52, 53
history taking 39
hypothesis 1, 2, 9, 10, 12, 13, 35, 36, 43, 45

ICMJE 3, 9, 25
IMRAD 2, 3, 38, 39, 41, 50
inclusion criteria 27

intensifiers 22
interventions 2, 9, 22, 38, 41, 44, 50, 51
introduction 2, 9–13, 17, 21, 22, 46, 47

limitations 10, 12, 13, 45

main outcome measures 50, 51
management and outcome 39, 40
manuscript submission 54–59
meta-analyses 1, 3, 51, 53
meta-textual expression 36
methods 2, 12, 16, 22, 23, 25–29, 32, 44, 47
modality (see also "verbs, modal")
 19–23, 53
MOOSE 3, 9

noun, epistemic 48
noun, evaluative 53

objective (see also "purpose") 10, 12, 50
observational studies 1, 3, 28, 53
open review 58
outcome (see also "main outcome
 measures") 9, 12, 36, 37, 40, 43, 51

passive voice 27, 28, 31–34, 37, 53
past tense 27, 28, 37, 44
patients 6, 12, 20, 47, 50, 51, 52
phrase, procedural 37
present tense 12, 36, 44, 50
pseudo-passive 33, 34
purpose (see also "objective") 1, 2, 3, 4,
 10, 11, 12, 13, 35

QUOROM 3, 9

rationale 9, 10, 12, 13
references (see also "citations") 10, 11,
 47, 55
results 2, 16, 20, 26, 29, 35–38, 47, 51
review articles 1, 2, 3, 9, 20, 51, 53

self-reference 31–34
setting 50, 51
shielding 21–23, 47, 57
STARD 3, 4, 9, 35, 48
statistical analysis 26–29, 49
STROBE 3, 9

tables 36, 40, 55
theme 1, 5, 6, 9, 33, 47, 48
title 2, 5–7, 49
title, compound 5
title, full sentence 5
title, nominal 5
title, question 5
toning down 21

Uniform Requirements 3, 9, 25, 35,
 49, 55

validity 25, 26, 29, 45
verbs, cognition activity 11
verbs, discourse activity 11
verbs, epistemic 21
verbs, methods 28
verbs, modal 19, 47, 53
verbs, procedural 28
verbs, real-world or experimental
 activity 11
verbs, semi-auxiliary 20